Introduction 2

   Exam Structure 2

   Eligibility Requirements 2

      License Requirement 2

      Education Requirement 3

      Experience Requirement 3

Introduction about Author 4

Your plan to get Success 5

WCC Exam Practice Test 1 7

   Test 1 Answer Key 34

WCC Exam Practice Test 2 51

   Test 2 Answer Key 77

Rewards.. 94

Introduction

The Wound Care Certification (WCC) exam, administered by the National Alliance of Wound Care and Ostomy (NAWCO), evaluates a candidate's expertise in managing wounds. This certification demonstrates advanced-level competency beyond a standard wound care license. Divided into four key areas, the exam assesses knowledge in patient and wound information, plan of care, legal considerations, and skin analysis. By covering topics like obtaining patient history, selecting appropriate treatment options, ensuring accurate documentation, and analyzing skin integrity, the WCC exam ensures that certified professionals possess the necessary theoretical and practical skills to provide optimal wound care management.

Exam Structure

The WCC exam contains 110 multiple-choice questions, 10 of which are unscored, and you will be given a time limit of 2 hours. The unscored questions are used to evaluate questions for future versions of the exam, and you will not know which questions are scored or unscored.

Eligibility Requirements

To be eligible for the exam, you must meet the following license, education, and experience requirements:

License Requirement

For the license requirement, you must hold any one of the following valid and unrestricted licenses:

- RN
- LPN/LVN
- NP
- PA
- PTA
- OT
- OTA
- MD
- DO
- DPM

Education Requirement

- You must graduate from a skin and wound management course that meets certification criteria
- You must hold a current and active CWOCN, CWON, CWCN, or CWS certification

Experience Requirement

- You must complete at least 120 hours of hands-on clinical training
- You must complete at least two years of full-time or four years of part-time experience with wound care, management, education, or research directly related to wound care

Introduction about Author

Hey there! I am the author of this book and I am a wound care specialist who is passionate in my field of work sincerely assisting new professionals to do their best in passing the Wound Care Certification (WCC) test. I have created two mock tests plus a study guide to be used as your guide to test preparation.

Every question is followed by an answer justification that delves deeper into the subject, thus giving you a deeper understanding of the concepts. And, hey, if you spot an error or an idea to improve it sounds good to me! Just tell me, and spot on am I going to rectify. I make it your success!

Please scan QR code below to contact me if you found any mistake,

Your plan to get Success

Day 1	Introduction to WCC Exam Content outline and structure of the exam
Day 2	Explore the Official NAWCO Website
Day 3	Read and Study the reference book **PDF** from WCC Exam's official website, WCC Candidate Handbook **(FREE)**
Day 4	Domain 1: Patient and Wound Information, Review each subdomain in detail
Day 5	Obtain patient history by applying procedural concepts, Analyze characteristics of wounds
Day 6	Identify the types, stage or grade, and probable etiology of wounds, Determine any indications of compromised healing of the wound
Day 7	Begin Practice Test 1 - Read, Answer, and Review Explanations (Q1 to 30)
Day 8	Begin Practice Test 2 - Read, Answer, and Review Explanations (Q1 to 30)
Day 9	Read and study the reference book **PDF** from WCC Exam's official website, Acute & Chronic Wounds, Current Management Concepts **(FREE)**
Day 10	Domain 2: Plan of Care, review each subdomain in detail focusing on wound care treatment, preparation, and management of the wound bed
Day 11	Verify the plan's effectiveness and recommend revisions that are appropriate
Day 12	Determine if nutritional intervention is needed, Determine the educational plan
Day 13	Determine if diagnostic testing and any subsequent actions are needed
Day 14	Mitigate risk factors by determining preventative strategies
Day 15	Begin Practice Test 1 - Read, Answer, and Review Explanations (Q31 to 73)
Day 16	Begin Practice Test 2 - Read, Answer, and Review Explanations (Q31 to 73)
Day 17	Read and study the reference book **PDF** from WCC Exam's official website, Clinical Guide to Skin and Wound Care, Seventh edition **(FREE)**
Day 18	Domain 3: Legal, Review each subdomain in detail
Day 19	Ensuring accurate documentation by applying legal and institutional guidelines
Day 20	Apply best practices and care standards
Day 21	Apply legal concepts to the wound care practice
Day 22	Begin Practice Test 1 - Read, Answer, and Review Explanations (Q74 to 89)
Day 23	Begin Practice Test 1 - Read, Answer, and Review Explanations (Q74 to 89)

Day 24	Read and study the reference book **PDF** from WCC Exam's official website, Wound Care, A Collaborative Practice Manual for Health Professionals **(FREE)**
Day 25	Domain 4: Skin, review each subdomain in detail focusing on analyzing skin integrity across the patient's lifespan, Describe the functions and structures of normal skin
Day 26	Differentiate treatment options for abnormal skin conditions, describe wound healing phases, Analyze the impact of circulatory and lymphatic systems on wound healing
Day 27	Begin Practice Test 1 - Read, Answer, and Review Explanations (Q90 to 110)
Day 28	Begin Practice Test 1 - Read, Answer, and Review Explanations (Q90 to 110)
Day 29	Recheck the mistakes of practice tests 1 and 2 (check correct answer and explanation)
Day 30	Revise Questions and Answer explanations of practice tests 1 and 2

WCC Exam Practice Test 1

Q1. During wound assessment, what is the primary purpose of obtaining a patient's medication history?

A. Assessing allergy risk.

B. Evaluating treatment compliance.

C. Identifying potential contraindications.

D. Determining wound healing trajectory.

Q2. To assess the risk of lower extremity arterial disease (LEAD), which aspect of the patient's history is the most relevant?

A. History of hypertension management.

B. Presence of lower extremity edema.

C. Previous surgical procedures.

D. Smoking/tobacco use history.

Q3. Which condition is most likely indicated by the pain pattern in a patient with chronic wounds who presents with pain exacerbated by activity and relieved by rest?

A. Venous insufficiency

B. Arterial insufficiency

C. Diabetic neuropathy

D. Pressure ulceration

Q4. What historical information would be most appropriate to assess risk factors if a diabetic patient complains of recurrent foot ulcers?

A. Recent travel history.

B. Family history of allergies.

C. Duration of diabetes and glucose control.

D. History of seasonal allergies.

Q5. Which interdisciplinary approach is most appropriate for managing a patient with venous insufficiency presents with lower extremity ulcers?

A. Referral to a nutritionist.

B. Collaboration with a vascular surgeon.

C. Consultation with an allergist.

D. Involvement of a physical therapist.

Q6. For a patient with neuropathy and brownish skin discoloration around the ankles, what advice should be provided?

A. use off-loading methods.

B. undergo ankle-brachial index testing.

C. perform daily foot inspections.

D. elevate feet above heart level.

Q7. To promote wound healing, what adjunctive therapy is indicated when a patient with a history of burns presents with a partial-thickness wound?

A. Application of hydrogel dressings

B. Utilization of negative pressure wound therapy

C. Administration of broad-spectrum antibiotics

D. Application of silver sulfadiazine cream

Q8. Which dietary factor should be assessed to address potential exacerbating factors in a patient with a history of venous ulcers experiencing worsening lower extremity edema?

A. Sodium intake

B. Fiber intake

C. Vitamin D levels

D. Carbohydrate consumption

Q9. In the comprehensive assessment of wounds, how does the use of pain questionnaires contribute?

A. By replacing subjective pain assessments.

B. By facilitating the documentation of treatment outcomes.

C. By identifying pain patterns and assisting in diagnostic formulation.

D. By standardizing pain management protocols.

Q10. What type of wound is likely present when signs of tunneling and undermining are observed in a patient with a traumatic wound?

A. Pressure injury

B. Surgical wound

C. Diabetic foot ulcer

D. Full-thickness wound

Q11. What type of dressing is most suitable for a postoperative patient with a wound infection producing purulent discharge?

A. Alginate dressing.

B. Foam dressing.

C. Hydrogel dressing.

D. Antimicrobial dressing.

Q12. What intervention is crucial for preventing infection and promoting healing, if a patient with a traumatic wound presents with exposed tendon tissue?

A. Applying a hydrocolloid dressing.

B. Irrigating the wound with saline.

C. Administering systemic antibiotics.

D. Performing primary closure of the wound.

Q13. Utilizing the body's enzymes, which method of wound debridement gradually breaks down necrotic tissue?

A. Mechanical debridement using sharp instruments

B. Enzymatic debridement employing specialized topical agents

C. Autolytic debridement through moisture-retentive dressings

D. Biosurgical debridement utilizing sterile maggots

Q14. For creating a moist wound environment conducive to healing, which type of wound dressing is specifically indicated for this purpose?

A. Hydrocolloids

B. Gauze

C. Film dressings

D. Hydrogels

Q15. What action is contraindicated in managing a wound with black necrotic tissue?

A. Applying hydrogel dressing

B. Performing sharp debridement

C. Administering antibiotics

D. Using autolytic debridement

Q16. What type of ulcer is most likely present when a patient with a history of leg swelling and varicose veins presents with non-healing wounds on the inner aspect of the lower leg, just above the ankle?

A. Lower Leg Ulcer

B. Diabetic Foot Ulcer

C. Venous Stasis Ulcer

D. Arterial (Ischemic) Ulcer

Q17. What is the most likely diagnosis, if a patient with sickle cell anemia presents with a non-healing wound on their foot?

A. Venous ulcer

B. Arterial ulcer

C. Diabetic foot ulcer

D. Osteomyelitis

Q18. In terms of their underlying causes and treatment modalities particularly, how radiation burns differ from other burn injuries?

A. Depth of tissue involvement

B. Presence of infection

C. Etiology

D. Requirement of surgical intervention

Q19. When resulting from a traumatic incident, what type of wound involves the separation of multiple layers of skin, commonly requiring careful suturing for adequate closure?

A. Skin laceration

B. Gangrenous wound

C. Skin tear

D. Radiation burn

Q20. What characteristic is indicative of wound infection when a patient presents with a wound showing signs of redness, heat, pain, and swelling?

A. Serous exudate

B. Clear exudate

C. Granulation tissue

D. Erythema and warmth

Q21. Considering traumatic wounds as a common type of acute injury, what primary factor contributes to their development?

A. Pressure ulcers caused by prolonged immobility or poor circulation

B. Venous insufficiency leading to tissue hypoxia and necrosis

C. Naturopathic factors such as environmental exposures or allergic reactions

D. Bone fractures and soft tissue injuries from accidents or physical trauma

Q22. What additional assessment is crucial to determine the etiology of the non-healing wound when a patient develops a wound over the sacrum with intact skin but nonblanchable redness, despite interventions?

A. Measurement of transcutaneous oxygen levels

B. Examination of capillary refill time

C. Assessment of nutritional status

D. Evaluation of blood pressure

Q23. In terms of wound characteristics, what sets apart venous ulcers from arterial ulcers?

A. Presence of slough.

B. Shiny wound bed appearance.

C. Irregular wound margins.

D. Association with distal extremity pain.

Q24. What might the healthcare provider explain about venous ulcers if a patient with a venous ulcer asks why their wound heals slower than others?

A. Decreased collagen synthesis

B. Reduced angiogenesis

C. Impaired macrophage activity

D. Altered TGFβ concentration

Q25. What type of growth factor is likely increased in the wound bed when a patient with chronic wounds shows signs of infection?

A. TGFβ

B. PDGF

C. EGF

D. VEGF

Q26. Which growth factor stimulates angiogenesis and promotes ingrowth of blood vessels during the proliferative phase of wound healing when a 65-year-old diabetic patient undergoes surgery for a foot wound?

A. Platelet-derived growth factor (PDGF)

B. Keratinocyte-derived growth factor (KGF)

C. Vascular endothelial growth factor (VEGF)

D. Basic fibroblast growth factor (bFGF)

Q27. During the inflammatory phase of wound healing, what is the primary function of platelets in initiating the coagulation cascade and promoting amplification and recruitment of cells for debridement?

A. Forming a platelet plug

B. Phagocytosis of dead tissue

C. Stimulation of angiogenesis

D. Production of cytokines

Q28. Which genetic disorder may cause delayed wound healing and keloid formation if a patient exhibits yellowish papules over flexure sites?

A. Pseudoxanthoma elasticum

B. Ehlers-Danlos syndrome

C. Cutis laxa

D. Marfan syndrome

Q29. By severely drooping skin folds, cardiovascular, and pulmonary comorbidities due to an inborn error in elastin, which derangement in wound healing is characterized?

A. Pseudoxanthoma elasticum

B. Ehlers-Danlos syndrome

C. Marfan syndrome

D. Cutis laxa

Q30. During the early inflammatory phase, what initiates the molecular events leading to the infiltration of neutrophils in the wound site?

A. Complement cascade activation

B. Macrophage secretion

C. Platelet aggregation

D. Fibroblast proliferation

Q31. What should be recommended to the patient with a stage 3 pressure ulcer on the sacrum?

A. Use a pressure-relieving mattress.

B. Apply topical antibiotics.

C. Keep the wound exposed to air.

D. Increase dietary fat intake.

Q32. What is the primary goal of wound care in the treatment of a patient with a chronic wound?

A. Increasing friction around the wound site.

B. Promoting a moist wound environment.

C. Applying harsh chemicals to the wound bed.

D. Exposing the wound to sunlight.

Q33. When selecting a wound dressing for a patient with a highly exudating wound, what is a crucial aspect to consider?

A. Choosing a dressing that promotes dryness.

B. Opting for a dressing that requires frequent changes.

C. Selecting a dressing that absorbs moisture effectively.

D. Using a dressing that adheres strongly to the wound bed.

Q34. What should be a primary consideration when developing a plan of care for a patient with limited financial resources?

A. Prescribing expensive wound care products.

B. Selecting treatments that are financially reasonable.

C. Ignoring the patient's financial constraints.

D. Recommending home remedies for wound care.

Q35. What should healthcare professionals prioritize regarding caregivers when considering wound care product selection?

A. Ignoring caregiver preferences.

B. Ensuring products are complex to use.

C. Accounting for caregiver skill level and concerns.

D. Selecting products based solely on cost-effectiveness.

Q36. What role do patient preferences play when developing a wound care plan?

A. Patient preferences are irrelevant in wound care planning.

B. Patient preferences should be considered alongside clinical guidelines.

C. Patient preferences should be prioritized over clinical recommendations.

D. Patient preferences should only be considered if they align with healthcare provider opinions.

Q37. In a patient with suspected arterial ulcers, which diagnostic test is recommended to assess arterial insufficiency?

A. Contrast venogram.

B. Air plethysmography.

C. Doppler ultrasonography.

D. Ankle-brachial index (ABI).

Q38. A healthcare provider suspects venous insufficiency in a patient with chronic leg ulcers. To confirm the diagnosis, what diagnostic test should be prioritized?

A. Contrast venogram.

B. Air plethysmography.

C. Doppler ultrasonography.

D. Ankle-brachial index (ABI).

Q39. Which diagnostic test is recommended to confirm arterial insufficiency through segmental pressure measurements in a patient with suspected arterial ulcers?

A. Doppler ultrasonography.

B. Ankle-brachial index (ABI).

C. Toe pressure measurements.

D. Segmental pressure measurements.

Q40. What does a toe pressure of less than 30 mm Hg indicate if a patient suspected of arterial insufficiency presents decreased toe pressure?

A. Poor healing potential.

B. Normal healing potential.

C. Adequate arterial perfusion.

D. Medial calcification of arteries.

Q41. What diagnostic test is measured using a laser Doppler flow sensor and provides information about post-occlusive reactive hyperemia?

A. Skin perfusion pressure assessment.

B. Transcutaneous oxygen measurements.

C. Toe-brachial index measurement.

D. Magnetic resonance angiography.

Q42. What is a notable disadvantage of contrast venogram compared to noninvasive methods in a patient with suspected arterial ulcers?

A. Limited accuracy in diagnosing arterial occlusion.

B. High sensitivity to arterial insufficiency.

C. Risk of local thrombophlebitis and deep vein thrombosis.

D. Inability to assess arterial waveforms.

Q43. Which nutrient deficiency may delay wound healing in a patient with poor nutritional intake who presents with a pressure ulcer?

A. Vitamin D

B. Vitamin C

C. Vitamin B12

D. Vitamin K

Q44. To reduce the incidence of pressure ulcers in at-risk patients, what is the recommended dietary supplement?

A. Vitamin D

B. Iron

C. Omega-3 fatty acids

D. Oral nutritional supplement

Q45. How do low serum protein levels contribute to the development of pressure ulcers in a patient with a pressure ulcer?

A. Increases oxygen diffusion

B. Enhances tissue regeneration

C. Decreases immune function

D. Promotes collagen synthesis

Q46. Which tool includes components like nutrition assessment and intervention and is considered the criterion standard for nutrition practice?

A. Subjective Global Assessment.

B. Resident Assessment Instrument.

C. Nutrition Care Process.

D. Comprehensive nutrition assessment.

Q47. Which intervention should be avoided to prevent disruption of normal phagocytic activity if a 70-year-old patient with a Stage III pressure ulcer presents with low serum zinc levels?

A. Zinc supplementation

B. Iron supplementation

C. Copper supplementation

D. Vitamin C supplementation

Q48. To enhance wound healing, what is the recommended duration for zinc supplementation in a patient with normal zinc levels having a chronic wound?

A. 1 to 2 weeks

B. 3 to 4 weeks

C. 5 to 6 weeks

D. 7 to 10 days

Q49. A patient's chronic wound with increased exudate, redness, and foul odor is assessed by a wound care nurse. What phase of wound bioburden is suggested by this presentation?

A. Contamination

B. Colonization

C. Critical colonization

D. Biofilm

Q50. A patient's chronic wound with increased exudate and odor is assessed by a wound care clinician. In this case, what is the primary objective of topical antimicrobial therapy?

A. Promote granulation tissue formation

B. Inhibit biofilm formation

C. Reduce wound exudate

D. Prevent microbial colonization

Q51. Which method selectively removes only necrotic tissue if a wound care clinician selects a debridement method for a necrotic wound?

A. Mechanical

B. Autolytic

C. Chemical

D. Biologic

Q52. What would be the primary benefit of debridement if a wound care specialist treats a chronic wound with necrotic tissue?

A. Reducing bacterial load

B. Stimulating healthy tissue growth

C. Enhancing moisture balance

D. Promoting epithelial advancement

Q53. Which antimicrobial agent is commonly used for its effectiveness against Staphylococcus aureus including MRSA when a patient with a chronic wound presents with heavy bacterial colonization?

A. Cetrimide-based cleansers

B. Mupirocin

C. Silver compounds

D. Iodine

Q54. What aspect of wound bed preparation is emphasized when a chronic wound fails to progress through the normal phases of healing?

A. Necrotic tissue removal

B. Moisture balance

C. Debridement frequency

D. Assessment of wound edges

Q55. In cases of deep partial-thickness burns, what is the most common surgical intervention for patients with burn injuries?

A. Application of topically applied growth factors

B. Bioengineered skin grafts

C. Negative pressure wound therapy

D. Electrical stimulation therapy

Q56. In what ways does wound bed preparation contribute to the effectiveness of advanced wound care therapies like topically applied growth factors?

A. Enhances the patient's comfort

B. Reduces treatment cost

C. Maximizes therapy benefits

D. Accelerates wound infection

Q57. A patient with a chronic wound has undergone HVPC wound treatment. After cleansing the wound thoroughly, what should be done to enhance electrical stimulation effectiveness?

A. Apply a dry gauze pad over the wound.

B. Debride necrotic tissue immediately.

C. Soak gauze pads in normal saline solution.

D. Leave the wound uncovered for air exposure.

Q58. What is emphasized regarding the routine use of antibiotics for all wounds in wound care management?

A. Essential for all wounds

B. Recommended for infected wounds

C. Discouraged unless signs of infection

D. Mandatory for chronic wounds

Q59. In diabetic patients, which of the following is the recommended approach to managing neuropathic ulcers that do not heal readily with off-loading, provided arterial blood supply is adequate?

A. Continuous antibiotic therapy

B. Application of hydrogel dressings

C. Excision of the entire ulcer bed

D. Routine debridement with a scalpel

Q60. What footwear recommendation promotes safety when a patient with diabetic neuropathy and limited mobility is at risk for foot ulcers?

A. Barefoot walking

B. Tight-fitting shoes

C. Sandals with arch support

D. Adjustable shoes with hook and loop closures

Q61. What contextual factors impact education in real-world settings, when a caregiver faces challenges in providing diabetes education due to time constraints and low reimbursement?

A. Physician knowledge

B. Practice economics

C. Patient attitude

D. Comprehensive programs

Q62. What should caregivers report to the healthcare provider when a patient with a malignant cutaneous wound experience severe emotional distress?

A. Changes in wound appearance

B. Increased pain

C. Malodorous exudates

D. All of the above

Q63. Before teaching pouching techniques, what factors should be considered when educating patients and caregivers about fistula management?

A. Patient's favorite color

B. Patient's shoe size

C. Patient's self-care ability

D. Patient's preferred hairstyle

Q64. When educating a burn patient about wound care, what aspect of dressing changes should be emphasized to improve prognosis?

A. Frequency of dressing changes

B. Type of bandaging

C. Importance of pain management

D. Schedule for a skin check

Q65. When educating a patient with a burn injury, what nutritional advice supports wound healing and improved activities of daily living?

A. Low fluid intake

B. High-quality protein

C. Excessive carbohydrates

D. Minimal dietary fat

Q66. Which of the following factors primarily affect the functional and cosmetic outcome of radiation skin reactions in patients receiving radiation therapy and at risk for severe skin reactions?

A. Patient's age and nutritional status

B. Treatment schedule and total dose

C. Use of concomitant chemotherapy

D. Moisture content of the treatment area

Q67. Which factor is associated with impaired wound healing and advanced glycosylation, when assessing a patient's risk for foot ulcers in diabetes?

A. Absent protective sensation

B. Autonomic neuropathy

C. Limited joint mobility

D. Impaired vision

Q68.A patient is at risk for lymphedema. The nurse should educate the patient on preventative strategies. In this case, what action helps reduce the patient's lymphedema risk?

A. Applying tight compression garments

B. Avoiding limb elevation

C. Exposing the affected area to extreme cold or heat

D. Taking good care of skin and nails

Q69. What should be included in education regarding skin checks to prevent complications when a caregiver is assisting a patient with burns in daily wound care?

A. Assessment of emotional distress

B. Identification of pressure points

C. Daily fluid intake monitoring

D. Selection of preferred dressing colors

Q70. How can healthcare professionals play a role in promoting tobacco cessation?

A. Encourage general stress management.

B. Recommend elevated homocysteine testing.

C. Prescribe antibiotics for infection.

D. Suggest avoiding compression stockings.

Q71. In the context of patient-provider contracts for tobacco cessation, what stands out as a crucial factor?

A. Commitment to hypertension management.

B. Setting a date to eliminate tobacco use.

C. Social isolation prevention.

D. Family history assessment.

Q72. What adult learning principles should be considered for effective education delivery when a wound specialist develops an educational plan for a burn patient?

A. Assessing caregiver's willingness to learn

B. Identifying patient's preferred dressing colors

C. Offering a one-time education session

D. Relying on the patient's past educational experiences

Q73. Among patients with wounds, what plays a pivotal role as a major risk factor for calf pump muscle dysfunction?

A. Sedentary lifestyle

B. Obesity

C. Leg trauma

D. Advanced age

Q74. There is a patient with multiple wounds. One wound in a cluster has already been healed. In this case, how should the nurse approach documentation for the remaining wounds?

A. Change reference names for all wounds in the cluster

B. Omit documentation for the healed wound

C. Retain the same reference names for all remaining wounds

D. Create a new medical record for each remaining wound

Q75. Which assessment tool is most suitable for a wound care clinician to monitor wound healing progress reliably without linear measurements?

A. Pressure Ulcer Scale for Healing (PUSH)

B. Visual Analog Scale (VAS)

C. Bates-Jensen Wound Assessment Tool (BWAT)

D. Wound Healing Tracking Tool (WHTT)

Q76. In the context of wound care documentation, how can wound photographs serve as a legal defense?

A. By showcasing clinician accomplishments

B. By providing a permanent record of the wound

C. By preventing the need for uniform terminology

D. By eliminating the need for written documentation

Q77. There is a patient with a Stage 2 Ulcer on the sacrum. In this situation, the patient should be advised to:

A. Use a donut-shaped cushion.

B. Avoid sitting for prolonged periods.

C. Apply antibiotic ointment daily.

D. Increase intake of vitamin C.

Q78. There is a patient with a diabetic foot ulcer. The patient requires documentation to promote healing. In this case, what should be included in the documentation?

A. Presence of induration

B. Dietary supplements and vitamins

C. Type and amount of wound exudate

D. Weekly skin reports

Q79. There is a resident in a long-term care facility. He is suspected to have a deep tissue injury. In this case, the nurse's initial action should be to:

A. Apply a transparent film dressing

B. Measure and document the ulcer's depth

C. Perform a bedside biopsy

D. Consult a wound care specialist

Q80. A patient with venous leg ulcers comes to the clinic. He experiences persistent pain and swelling. The nurse should:

A. Apply warm compresses

B. Elevate the legs above heart level

C. Encourage vigorous exercise

D. Apply compression therapy

Q81. What patient-based variables should a wound care provider prioritize for documentation when assessing a patient's wound?

A. Wound size changes

B. Type of dressing used

C. Temperature of the room

D. Time of the last medication administration

Q82. There is a patient with a non-healing wound. The patient presents with signs of biofilm after two weeks of standard care. In this case, what is the most aggressive debridement method to combat biofilm?

A. Autolytic debridement

B. Enzymatic debridement

C. Mechanical debridement

D. Sharp debridement

Q83. After two weeks of standard care, a patient's wound fails to show improvement. In this case, what should be the next step according to wound care standards?

A. Reconsider the treatment plan

B. Increase frequency of dressing changes

C. Consult with a wound care specialist

D. Initiate advanced wound therapies

Q84. During the implementation of guidelines, what role did the wound care program manager play in supporting local committee chairs?

A. Strict enforcer of guidelines

B. Ignored local committee chairs

C. Provided situational leadership by supporting, coaching, and delegating

D. Relying solely on centralized decisions

Q85. In the context of deployment phase of the wound care program, what was the primary purpose of the executive steering group?

A. Enforcing guidelines uniformly

B. Considering site-specific implementation needs and variations

C. Ignoring local circumstances

D. Restricting the adaptation of guidelines

Q86. In what ways did the wound care program ensure the spread of guidelines, considering different levels of complexity?

A. Ignoring complexity levels.

B. Developing a one-size-fits-all approach.

C. Using a two-pronged approach involving communication and education based on complexity.

D. Relying solely on centralized decisions.

Q87. Which legal defense is invoked when a physician sutures a wound but leaves the bedside, resulting in a patient fall and injury?

A. Contributory negligence

B. Assumption of risk

C. Good Samaritan

D. Sudden emergency

Q88. What should be done to minimize legal risk when managing wounds with potential foreign bodies?

A. Advise strict bed rest

B. Perform radiographs routinely

C. Prescribe prophylactic antibiotics

D. Document thorough examination and warnings

Q89. What advice should the clinician give to a patient whose wound examination yields no foreign body but whose persistent pain prompts a return visit?

A. Disregard the pain unless it worsens

B. Document symptoms and discharge the patient

C. Perform immediate exploratory surgery

D. Warn of potential retained foreign body and instruct on return criteria

Q90. When a patient with a stage 2 pressure ulcer on the sacrum complains of pain. The nurse's priority intervention is to:

A. Apply a hydrocolloid dressing.

B. Administer oral analgesics.

C. Re-position the patient every 2 hours.

D. Consult a wound care specialist.

Q91. What initial action should the clinician take when a diabetic patient, with a foot wound, presents with signs of infection?

A. Order a broad-spectrum antibiotic.

B. Refer for surgical debridement.

C. Perform a thorough wound assessment.

D. Apply a moist wound dressing.

Q92. What should be the appropriate wound classification for a patient with diabetes and altered skin integrity, presenting with erythema and partial skin thickness loss?

A. Stage 1

B. Stage 2

C. Stage 3

D. Stage 4

Q93. In a bedridden patient, a caregiver notices skin discoloration and firmness. What intrinsic factor should be considered in the skin assessment?

A. Falls

B. Diabetes

C. Accidents

D. Immobility

Q94. What medication class is most likely contributing to skin damage when an elderly patient is hospitalized with impaired skin integrity?

A. Antibiotics

B. Thyroid hormones

C. Insulin

D. Nonsteroidal anti-inflammatory drugs (NSAIDs)

Q95. When a clinician notices overexposure to moisture in a patient's wound. What potential impact on skin integrity should be considered?

A. Improved blood flow

B. Enhanced cell metabolism

C. Disruption of the skin barrier

D. Accelerated tissue regeneration

Q96. In maintaining skin integrity, what is the primary function of the epidermis?

A. Regulating body temperature

B. Providing a physical barrier

C. Synthesizing collagen

D. Facilitating blood circulation

Q97. A patient with dry, flaky skin and increased transepidermal water loss may benefit from interventions aimed at:

A. increasing ceramide synthesis.

B. reducing cholesterol synthesis.

C. limiting fatty acid production.

D. avoiding topical moisturizers.

Q98. In maintaining skin integrity, what is the primary function of the stratum corneum?

A. Producing melanocytes for pigmentation.

B. Regulating thermoregulation through sweat.

C. Providing resistance to pathogenic organisms.

D. Synthesizing collagen for skin strength.

Q99. When a patient presents with chronic leg ulcers, peripheral neuropathy, and brownish skin discoloration. The optimal treatment strategy for preventing complications involves:

A. Compression therapy.

B. Immobilization in a cast.

C. Topical antimicrobial agents.

D. Hyperbaric oxygen therapy.

Q100. A diabetic patient with Charcot arthropathy and peripheral neuropathy seeks wound care advice. The most appropriate noninvasive intervention to support bone healing is:

A. Electrostimulation.

B. Compression bandages.

C. Topical corticosteroids.

D. Pamidronate administration.

Q101. What should be the initial intervention when a patient with a non-healing diabetic foot ulcer exhibits signs of infection, including increased exudate and erythema?

A. Apply a topical growth factor.

B. Perform surgical debridement.

C. Administer systemic antibiotics.

D. Use negative pressure wound therapy.

Q102. For surgical excision and skin grafting, a burn patient with extensive full-thickness wounds is scheduled. What is the appropriate topical agent for preoperative wound management?

A. Hydrogel dressings

B. Silver sulfadiazine cream

C. Moisturizer application

D. Antimicrobial ointment

Q103. In the context of wound healing, what is the likely consequence of delay when a patient with a surgical wound healing by primary intention experiences prolonged inflammation?

A. Faster tissue regeneration

B. Increased risk of infection

C. Accelerated maturation phase

D. Reduced scarring

Q104. Which phase of wound healing is primarily responsible for the symptoms where a wound care nurse notices signs of inflammation around a patient's wound, including redness, heat, swelling, and pain?

A. Maturation

B. Proliferation

C. Inflammation

D. Destruction

Q105. In wound healing, what is the consequence of localized ischemia in a patient with prolonged inflammation in a wound?

A. Accelerated epithelial proliferation

B. Reduced risk of infection

C. Increased damage to cell membranes

D. Enhanced synthesis of collagen

Q106. Which cell types play a crucial role in supporting capillary growth, collagen formation, and granulation tissue development, during the proliferative phase of wound healing?

A. Neutrophils

B. Macrophages

C. Fibroblasts and endothelial cells

D. T-lymphocytes

Q107. What condition is likely to hinder wound healing when a patient with diabetes and impaired vascular flow presents a chronic wound with measured tissue oxygen tensions at 15 mm Hg?

A. Hyperoxia

B. Hypoxia

C. Anemia

D. Edema

Q108. In wound healing, what is the role of lymphangiogenesis?

A. Facilitates tissue edema

B. Delays inflammation resolution

C. Drains fluids and activates immune responses

D. Promotes chronic inflammation

Q109. What abnormality is observed in inflammatory cell function in diabetic wound healing, contributing to reduced lymphatic structures in granulation tissue and impaired healing?

A. Increased macrophage number

B. Prolonged inflammatory phase

C. Elevated cytokine secretion

D. Enhanced VEGF release

Q110. What cardiovascular condition disrupts normal heart functioning, decreasing perfusion, delaying wound healing, and leading to compromised blood supply?

A. Peripheral vascular disease (PAD)

B. Congestive cardiac failure

C. Coronary artery disease (CAD)

D. Atherosclerosis

Test 1 Answer Key

Q1.

Answer: C

Explanation: Potential contraindications, interactions, and their influence on wound healing are determined by identifying medications, which guides treatment decisions.

Q2.

Answer: D

Explanation: When assessing vascular health and wound healing potential, the historical use of smoking/tobacco is imperative as it is a major risk factor for LEAD.

Q3.

Answer: B.

Explanation: Arterial insufficiency is indicated by this pain pattern, where activity increases the demand for blood flow, exacerbating the pain. Relief of symptoms during rest further indicates ischemia.

Q4.

Answer: C.

Explanation: In diabetic patients, assessing the duration of diabetes and glucose control are essential for evaluating the risk of foot ulcers, which highlights the significance of glycemic management in wound care.

Q5.

Answer: D.

Explanation: Management of venous insufficiency and its associated ulcers requires the involvement of a physical therapist, who can offer interventions such as compression therapy and exercise programs.

Q6.

Answer: C

Explanation: Neuropathic patients require regular foot checks to catch foot ulcers or injuries early, which are vital for preventing complications. These inspections are important to reduce the risk of severe problems and maintain foot health.

Q7.

Answer: B

Explanation: By enhancing tissue perfusion, reducing edema, and promoting granulation tissue formation, negative pressure wound therapy promotes wound healing, facilitating wound closure and healing.

Q8.

Answer: A

Explanation: Managing edema associated with venous ulcers necessitates assessing sodium intake because excessive sodium can increase fluid retention, exacerbating ulceration and edema.

Q9.

Answer: C.

Explanation: Tailoring appropriate pain management strategies and wound care plans is supported by structured pain questionnaires, which provide structured data regarding the nature, intensity, and localization of pain.

Q10.

Answer: D.

Explanation: Full-thickness wounds, characterized by tunneling and undermining, extend through the dermis and may involve deeper structures.

Q11.

Answer: D.

Explanation: While Alginate, foam, and hydrogel dressings are more suitable for different wound types, an antimicrobial dressing is specially designed to combat infection and aids in healing wounds with purulent discharge.

Q12.

Answer: B.

Explanation: For preventing infection and promoting healing, it is crucial to irrigate the wound with saline, which helps remove debris and reduce bacterial load. Dressings and antibiotics alone won't address wound cleanliness.

Q13.

Answer: C

Explanation: For breaking down necrotic tissue, autolytic debridement utilizes moisture-retentive dressings to facilitate the body's enzymes.

Q14.

Answer: D

Explanation: Recommended for their capacity to create and maintain a moist wound environment, hydrogels promote optimal healing conditions.

Q15.

Answer: B

Explanation: If vascular insufficiency is suspected sharp debridement is contraindicated as it may cause tissue damage.

Q16.

Answer: C

Explanation: Due to poor circulation, Venous Stasis Ulcers are typically present on the lower leg, above the ankle, in individuals with venous insufficiency.

Q17.

Answer: D

Explanation: Impaired blood flow in patients with sickle cell anemia increases the risk of developing osteomyelitis, resulting in non-healing wounds often seen in the feet.

Q18.

Answer: C

Explanation: Distinguishing them in etiology from other types of burns, radiation burns originate from radiation exposure frequently in the context of cancer treatment.

Q19.

Answer: A

Explanation: Necessitating sutures for healing, skin lacerations entail torn and ragged wounds that penetrate deep layers of skin.

Q20.

Answer: D

Explanation: The cardinal signs of inflammation like erythema, heat, pain, and swelling signify wound infection, arising from the body's immune response to combat pathogens, mandating prompt treatment for optimal healing.

Q21.

Answer: D

Explanation: Representing an acute type of injury, traumatic wounds are typically caused by accidents or injuries, involving bone fractures or soft tissue damage.

Q22.

Answer: A

Explanation: Understanding tissue perfusion and determining the contribution of ischemia to the non-healing wound can be facilitated by measuring transcutaneous oxygen levels.

Q23.

Answer: C.

Explanation: The underlying causes and vascular conditions are differentiated by the irregular margins of venous ulcers and well-defined edges of arterial ulcers, which aid in diagnosis and treatment.

Q24.

Answer: B.

Explanation: Due to chronic venous insufficiency, venous ulcers often exhibit impaired angiogenesis and delay wound healing by hindering the formation of new blood vessels.

Q25.

Answer: A.

Explanation: An increase in TGFβ levels following infection modulates the inflammatory response to aid wound healing and promotes tissue repair.

Q26.

Answer: C

Explanation: During the proliferative phase of wound healing, endothelial cells produce vascular endothelial growth factor (VEGF) that promotes angiogenesis.

Q27.

Answer: A

Explanation: Marking the onset of the inflammatory phase, wound healing is initiated through platelets by forming a platelet plug that limits bleeding, initiates the coagulation cascade, and promotes the recruitment of cells for debridement.

Q28.

Answer: A

Explanation: Yellowish papules characterize pseudoxanthoma elasticum and are linked with the formation of keloid and delayed wound healing.

Q29.

Answer: D.

Explanation: The presence of loose, drooping skin folds and associated cardiovascular and pulmonary complications suggests cutis laxa resulting from elastin deficiency and reflects impaired wound healing.

Q30.

Answer: A

Explanation: Neutrophil infiltration in the wound site during the early inflammatory phase is initiated by the activation of the complement cascade, leading to the molecular events.

Q31.

Answer: A

Explanation: Using pressure-relieving mattresses aids in wound healing, prevents further damage and helps alleviate pressure on vulnerable areas.

Q32.

Answer: B

Explanation: Promoting a moist wound environment promotes efficient healing and supports cellular migration.

Q33.

Answer: C

Explanation: A dressing that absorbs moisture, maintains a moist wound environment conducive to healing and effectively helps in managing exudate.

Q34.

Answer: B

Explanation: Selecting financially reasonable treatments facilitates a sustainable plan of care and promotes patient adherence.

Q35.

Answer: C

Explanation: Prioritizing caregiver skill levels and concerns is crucial for enhancing adherence and improving patient outcomes in wound care product selection.

Q36.

Answer: B

Explanation: A comprehensive approach to wound care planning that respects individual needs and preferences is ensured by integrating patient preferences alongside clinical guidelines.

Q37.

Answer: D

Explanation: To assess arterial insufficiency and guide wound care management in patients with suspected arterial ulcers, an Ankle-brachial index (ABI) is used which is a simple and noninvasive test.

Q38.

Answer: C

Explanation: Doppler ultrasonography is noninvasive and aids in the diagnosis of venous insufficiency, providing valuable information about venous reflux.

Q39.

Answer: D

Explanation: Crucial information about arterial insufficiency is provided by segmental pressure. A drop of more than 20 to 30 mm Hg indicates arterial occlusion.

Q40.

Answer: A

Explanation: Due to inadequate arterial perfusion, a toe pressure of less than 30 mm Hg indicates poor healing potential.

Q41.

Answer: A

Explanation: By using a laser Doppler flow sensor, skin perfusion pressure assessment measures post-occlusive reactive hyperemia. This aids in assessing perfusion adequacy.

Q42.

Answer: C

Explanation: A risk of inducing local thrombophlebitis and deep vein thrombosis is carried by a Contrast venogram. This makes it less desirable than noninvasive methods.

Q43.

Answer: B

Explanation: By impairing collagen synthesis and immune function, vitamin C deficiency delays wound healing.

Q44.

Answer: D

Explanation: In at-risk patients, the incidence of pressure ulcer development is significantly reduced by oral nutritional supplements.

Q45.

Answer: C

Explanation: Immune function is decreased by low serum protein levels. This makes tissues more susceptible to breakdown and pressure ulcer development.

Q46.

Answer: C

Explanation: The Nutrition Care Process is considered the criterion standard for nutrition practice including components like nutrition assessment and intervention.

Q47.

Answer: A

Explanation: Excessive zinc supplementation may weaken scar tissue, disrupt normal phagocytic activity and lead to copper deficiency.

Q48.

Answer: D

Explanation: To avoid potential disruptions in normal phagocytic activity, supplementation should be limited to 7 to 10 days for patients with normal zinc levels.

Q49.

Answer: C

Explanation: Critical colonization is suggested by the NERDS signs—nonhealing, increased exudate, redness, debris, and smell. This requires topical antimicrobial treatment.

Q50.

Answer: B

Explanation: The objective of topical antimicrobials is to eradicate pathogenic microorganisms and inhibit biofilm formation which contributes to effective wound management.

Q51.

Answer: B

Explanation: Necrotic tissue is removed by Autolytic debridement. This aids in wound healing by promoting the natural enzymatic breakdown of devitalized tissue.

Q52.

Answer: B

Explanation: Debridement facilitates a stimulatory environment for healthy tissue growth and wound healing and removes necrotic tissue.

Q53.

Answer: C

Explanation: In wound management, silver compounds are effective against Staphylococcus aureus including MRSA such as silver sulphadiazine.

Q54.

Answer: A

Explanation: To address the failure of wounds to progress through normal healing phases, necrotic tissue removal is emphasized which is a key of wound bed preparation.

Q55.

Answer: B

Explanation: Bioengineered skin grafts are the most common surgical intervention for such burns when a patient with a burn injury has deep partial-thickness wounds.

Q56.

Answer: C

Explanation: Adequate wound bed preparation ensures the wound is infection-free, well-vascularized, and devoid of scarring. It optimizes the effectiveness of advanced therapies like topically applied growth factors.

Q57.

Answer: C

Explanation: Before applying soaking gauze pads in the normal saline solution helps create a conducive environment for HVPC wound treatment.

Q58.

Answer: C

Explanation: In wound care management, emphasis is placed on discouraging the routine use of antibiotics for all wounds unless signs of infection are present.

Q59.

Answer: C

Explanation: In diabetic patients, neuropathic ulcers that do not heal with offloading can be managed by excision of the entire ulcer bed, especially when the arterial blood supply is adequate.

Q60.

Answer: D

Explanation: Adjustable shoes with hook and loop closures promote safety when a patient with diabetic neuropathy and limited mobility is at risk for foot ulcers.

Q61.

Answer: B

Explanation: In real-world settings, time constraints and economic factors affect the delivery of diabetes education. They impact both patients and providers in operational settings

Q62.

Answer: D

Explanation: To ensure comprehensive care for patients with malignant cutaneous wounds, caregivers must report various conditions, including emotional distress, to the healthcare provider

Q63.

Answer: C

Explanation: Before teaching poaching techniques, considering the patient's self-care ability is crucial when educating patients and caregivers about fistula management. This ensures tailored education and effective care strategies.

Q64.

Answer: A

Explanation: For optimal wound care, emphasizing the frequency of dressing changes is crucial, affecting prognosis and overall healing outcomes.

Q65.

Answer: B

Explanation: For wound healing and improved activities of daily living in burn patients, high-quality protein is essential as it promotes optimal recovery.

Q66.

Answer: B

Explanation: The treatment schedule and total dose primarily affect the functional and cosmetic outcome of radiation-induced skin reactions.

Q67.

Answer: C

Explanation: Limited joint mobility contributes to impaired wound healing and advanced glycosylation. It is a risk factor for foot ulcers in diabetes.

Q68.

Answer: D

Explanation: The nurse should advise the patient to take good care of skin and nails. Good skin and nail care reduces the risk of lymphedema in at-risk patients.

Q69.

Answer: B

Explanation: Identification of pressure points should be included in education regarding skin checks to prevent complications in patients with burns. This approach promotes comprehensive wound care.

Q70.

Answer: A

Explanation: Healthcare professionals play a role in promoting tobacco cessation by encouraging stress management. Encouraging stress management is crucial for tobacco cessation as it helps patients cope without resorting to smoking during challenging situations.

Q71.

Answer: B

Explanation: Committing to a specific date for eliminating tobacco use and providing a clear goal and timeline for cessation is involved in the Patient–provider contracts.

Q72.

Answer: A

Explanation: "Assessing the caregiver's willingness to learn" is the principle that should be considered for effective education delivery. This principle ensures tailored and effective education for patients with burns.

Q73.

Answer: A

Explanation: Prolonged standing and a sedentary lifestyle contribute to calf pump muscle dysfunction in wound patients. It impacts venous return and perfusion.

Q74.

Answer: C

Explanation: The nurse should retain the same reference names for all remaining wounds. This approach ensures consistency and accurate documentation, allowing for effective tracking of each wound's progress.

Q75.

Answer: A

Explanation: The clinician should use the Pressure Ulcer Scale for Healing (PUSH) tool. This tool provides reliable tracking of wound healing without requiring linear measurements.

Q76.

Answer: B

Explanation: Wound photographs provide a permanent record of the wound. These photographs prevent litigation by providing visual evidence of the wound's baseline and progression throughout the patient's care.

Q77.

Answer: B

Explanation: In this condition, the patient should avoid sitting for prolonged periods. This will reduce the pressure on the sacrum and help prevent pressure ulcer progression.

Q78.

Answer: B

Explanation: Dietary supplements and vitamins should be included in the documentation for a patient with a diabetic foot ulcer. These are crucial for a comprehensive understanding of interventions promoting diabetic foot ulcer healing.

Q79.

Answer: B

Explanation: The nurse should measure and document the ulcer's depth. Accurate measurement guides appropriate interventions for deep tissue injuries by determining their depth and severity.

Q80.

Answer: D

Explanation: The nurse should apply compression therapy to this patient. Compression therapy helps reduce swelling and pain in venous leg ulcers by improving venous return and promoting healing.

Q81.

Answer: A

Explanation: Documenting changes in wound size provides valuable information about the healing process and guides adjustments in the treatment plan. It is crucial for tracking progress and determining the effectiveness of the wound care interventions.

Q82.

Answer: D

Explanation: Sharp debridement provides effective removal of necrotic tissue and debris. It is the most aggressive method to combat biofilm in chronic wounds.

Q83.

Answer: A

Explanation: It's crucial to reassess and potentially revise the treatment plan if a wound shows no improvement after two weeks.

Q84.

Answer: C

Explanation: During the implementation of guidelines, the program manager provided situational leadership, supporting, coaching, and delegating based on the needs of local committee chairs.

Q85.

Answer: B

Explanation: The primary purpose of the executive steering group was to consider site-specific needs and variations. This approach enhances the adaptability and effectiveness of guidelines at the local level.

Q86.

Answer: C

Explanation: The wound care program uses a two-pronged approach involving communication and education based on complexity. This approach ensures the effective spread of guidelines across different levels.

Q87.

Answer: D

Explanation: A sudden emergency is invoked when a physician sutures a wound but leaves the bedside, resulting in a patient fall and injury. The sudden emergency defense absolves the physician, acknowledging the unforeseen circumstances of the patient's fall.

Q88.

Answer: D

Explanation: In cases of retained foreign bodies, comprehensive documentation of examination and warnings mitigates legal risk.

Q89.

Answer: D

Explanation: The clinician should warn the patient of potential retained foreign bodies and instruct on return criteria. This approach ensures informed care and legal protection.

Q90.

Answer: C

Explanation: Regular repositioning is crucial in preventing and managing pressure ulcers, and it helps address the patient's pain.

Q91.

Answer: C

Explanation: To determine the extent of infection and guide appropriate interventions, including potential antibiotic use, it is crucial to conduct a comprehensive wound assessment.

Q92.

Answer: B

Explanation: For a patient with diabetes and altered skin integrity presenting with erythema and partial skin thickness loss, the appropriate wound classification is Stage 2.

Q93.

Answer: B

Explanation: When a caregiver notices skin discoloration and firmness in a bedridden patient, diabetes should be considered as an intrinsic factor in the skin assessment.

Q94.

Answer: A

Explanation: Antibiotics medication class is most likely contributing to skin damage when an elderly patient is hospitalized with impaired skin integrity.

Q95.

Answer: C

Explanation: When a clinician notices overexposure to moisture in a patient's wound, one should consider the potential impact on skin integrity, specifically the disruption of the skin barrier.

Q96.

Answer: B

Explanation: The primary function of the epidermis in maintaining skin integrity is to provide a vital physical barrier against microorganisms, chemicals, and environmental pollutants.

Q97.

Answer: A

Explanation: Promoting ceramide synthesis is crucial to addressing compromised skin barriers. Ceramides restore the lipid barrier, preventing water loss, and improving hydration in conditions with a compromised stratum corneum, such as dry, flaky skin.

Q98.

Answer: C

Explanation: Providing resistance to pathogenic organisms is the primary function of the stratum corneum in maintaining skin integrity. The stratum corneum acts as a vital physical barrier, maintaining skin integrity by resisting pathogenic organisms.

Q99.

Answer: A

Explanation: For managing chronic leg ulcers, promoting venous return, and preventing complications like infection and skin breakdown, compression therapy is essential.

Q100.

Answer: A

Explanation: The most appropriate noninvasive intervention to support bone healing is electrostimulation. It serves as an adjunctive treatment for Charcot arthropathy, enhancing bone healing.

Q101.

Answer: C

Explanation: When a patient with a non-healing diabetic foot ulcer exhibits signs of infection, including increased exudate and erythema, the initial intervention should be administering systemic antibiotics. It is a crucial factor in non-healing wounds.

Q102.

Answer: B

Explanation: When a burn patient with extensive full-thickness wounds is scheduled for surgical excision and skin grafting silver, sulfadiazine cream is the appropriate topical agent for preoperative wound management.

Q103.

Answer: B

Explanation: When a patient with a surgical wound healing by primary intention experiences prolonged inflammation, an increased risk of infection is likely a consequence of the delay in wound healing.

Q104.

Answer: C

Explanation: Inflammation in the wound healing process is primarily responsible for signs noticed by a wound care nurse, such as redness, heat, swelling, and pain around a patient's wound.

Q105.

Answer: C

Explanation: Increased damage to cell membranes is the consequence of ischemia in wound healing when a patient with prolonged inflammation in a wound experiences localized ischemia.

Q106.

Answer: C

Explanation: During the proliferative phase of wound healing, fibroblasts and endothelial cells play a crucial role in supporting capillary growth, collagen formation, and granulation tissue development.

Q107.

Answer: B

Explanation: In a patient with diabetes and impaired vascular flow, hypoxia is likely to hinder wound healing in a chronic wound with measured tissue oxygen tensions at 15 mm Hg.

Q108.

Answer: C

Explanation: By aiding in fluid drainage and activating immune responses through the transport of cells, lymphangiogenesis plays a crucial role in wound healing.

Q109.

Answer: B

Explanation: Diabetic wound healing exhibits a prolonged inflammatory phase in inflammatory cell function, contributing to reduced lymphatic structures in granulation tissue and impaired healing.

Q110.

Answer: B

Explanation: Congestive cardiac failure disrupts normal heart function, causing decreased perfusion, delaying wound healing, and compromising blood supply.

WCC Exam Practice Test 2

Q1. The wound care provider suspect's arterial insufficiency in a 45-year-old patient with a history of peripheral artery disease (PAD) and presents with a non-healing foot ulcer. What additional diagnostic test should be performed to confirm this suspicion?

A. Magnetic resonance angiography (MRA).

B. Transcutaneous oxygen measurement.

C. Skin biopsy.

D. Contrast arteriography.

Q2. What assessment is essential to evaluate vascular status if a patient with diabetes presents with a chronic foot wound?

A. Performing the Allen's test.

B. Evaluating pedal pulses.

C. Measuring the ankle-brachial index (ABI).

D. Conducting a capillary refill test.

Q3. What dietary recommendation would best support wound healing for a patient with diabetes presenting lower extremity ulcers?

A. Low-carbohydrate diet

B. High-protein diet

C. High-fat diet

D. Low-sodium diet

Q4. Which aspect of the patient's history need to be carefully consideration before initiating compression therapy, if an elderly patient with a history of cardiovascular disease presents with a chronic wound?

A. Past surgical procedures.

B. Current medication regimen.

C. Allergy to latex.

D. Cardiac history and signs of heart failure.

Q5. What interdisciplinary approach should the wound care provider take to address a 55-year-old patient with a diabetic foot ulcer who presents with signs of malnutrition?

A. Initiate aggressive wound debridement.

B. Refer the patient for psychological counseling.

C. Collaborate with a registered dietitian for nutritional assessment and intervention.

D. Increase the frequency of wound care visits.

Q6. For preventing foot ulceration in diabetic patients, which dietary factor is essential?

A. Carbohydrate intake

B. Sodium restriction

C. Protein consumption

D. Vitamin supplementation

Q7. What nutritional factor should be evaluated to optimize wound healing when a patient with a history of surgical wounds presents with wound dehiscence?

A. Iron levels

B. Vitamin C intake

C. Calcium supplementation

D. Zinc intake

Q8. What initial step is essential for assessing the nature and severity of pain when a patient with a diabetic foot ulcer reports persistent pain?

A. Utilize a pain questionnaire

B. Prescribe opioid analgesics

C. Recommend physical therapy

D. Perform a visual inspection

Q9. Which element of the patient history is particularly instrumental in guiding clinical evaluation and management decisions within the assessment of patients with swollen limbs?

A. Sociodemographic profile.

B. Psychological predispositions.

C. Chief complaints and medical history.

D. Cultural background and beliefs.

Q10. What is the most appropriate next step in wound management when a patient with a Stage 4 pressure injury presents with exposed bone and tendon?

A. Apply a hydrogel dressing

B. Perform surgical debridement

C. Initiate negative pressure wound therapy

D. Apply a silver-impregnated dressing

Q11. Which diagnosis indicates arterial insufficiency if a patient with a chronic wound is found to have peripheral artery disease?

A. Pale, cool skin

B. Edematous extremities

C. Increased granulation tissue

D. Warm, erythematous skin

Q12. What intervention is essential for promoting debridement when a patient with a pressure ulcer who presents with blackened necrotic tissue?

A. Topical silver application.

B. Enzymatic debriding agent.

C. Hyperbaric oxygen therapy.

D. Moist wound healing approach.

Q13. While facilitating the healing process, which category of wound dressings is specifically designed to promote a moist wound environment?

A. Traditional gauze dressings

B. Hydrocolloid dressings

C. Alginate dressings

D. Silicone-based dressings

Q14. In preventing hindrance of the healing process, what intervention is recommended for wounds with excessive exudate?

A. Applying compression therapy

B. Keeping the wound environment moist

C. Providing offloading methods

D. Controlling the drainage

Q15. What should be the initial step in wound management when a patient presents with a wound showing yellowish dead tissue?

A. Apply a film dressing.

B. Perform mechanical debridement.

C. Administer antibiotics.

D. Apply a hydrogel dressing.

Q16. What type of ulceration is likely to present if a patient complains of persistent pain in the feet, especially at night, with wounds typically located on pressure points?

A. Arterial (Ischemic) Ulcers

B. Diabetic Foot Ulcers

C. Venous Stasis Ulcers

D. Bone Infection

Q17. What type of wound is most likely present for a palliative care patient who presents with a non-healing wound resulting from prolonged moisture exposure due to urinary incontinence?

A. Venous ulcer

B. Arterial ulcer

C. Moisture-associated skin damage (MASD)

D. Diabetic foot ulcer

Q18. Which crucial stage involves the synthesis and deposition of essential extracellular matrix proteins in the tissue repair process?

A. Angiogenesis

B. Fibroplasia

C. Inflammation

D. Epithelialization

Q19. Characterized by tissue necrosis and inadequate blood supply, which underlying condition is most frequently associated with the development of gangrene?

A. High dietary fat intake

B. Insufficient blood flow

C. Excessive physical activity

D. Overuse of topical antibiotics

Q20. What classification does a wound belong to when it results from a traumatic injury that disrupts normal tissue architecture and fails to heal within the expected timeframe?

A. Acute wound

B. Chronic wound

C. Complicated wound

D. Traumatic wound

Q21. Which type of wound involves a loss of tissue with the skin remaining intact, according to wound classification criteria?

A. Closed wound

B. Open wound

C. Contaminated wound

D. Septic wound

Q22. What additional assessment is crucial to determine the depth and extent of tissue involvement when a patient with a stage 2 pressure ulcer on the sacrum complains of pain and tenderness in the area?

A. Digital palpation of the wound bed

B. Measurement of wound circumference

C. Assessment of peripheral neuropathy

D. Evaluation of systemic inflammatory markers

Q23. When considering their causative mechanisms, how do shear injuries predominantly manifest?

A. Gravity-induced tissue displacement

B. Excessive friction along skin surfaces

C. Prolonged pressure exerted on bony prominences

D. Restricted mobility leading to tissue ischemia

Q24. What fetal wound healing characteristic should be explained when a pregnant woman with a deep laceration asks why her wound heals differently?

A. Increased neutrophil count

B. Scar formation

C. Greater fibrosis

D. Rich extracellular matrix in HA

Q25. What is important during the maturation phase if a patient with a pressure injury asks about factors influencing wound strength?

A. Collagen type III secretion

B. Angiogenesis rate

C. Fibroblast proliferation

D. Macrophage remodeling

Q26. Which cell type is primarily responsible for debridement during the inflammatory phase of wound healing, if a 50-year-old male patient has a deep wound on his leg after a motorcycle accident?

A. Neutrophils

B. Macrophages

C. Platelets

D. Fibroblasts

Q27. During the inflammatory phase of wound healing, which cytokine is primarily released by neutrophils and acts as a both proinflammatory cytokine and a stimulus for keratinocyte proliferation?

A. Interleukin

B. Transforming growth factor beta (TGF-b)

C. Platelet-derived growth factor (PDGF)

D. Vascular endothelial growth factor (VEGF)

Q28. What is a common characteristic affecting wound healing in a patient with Ehlers-Danlos syndrome?

A. Hyperelastic skin

B. Hypermobile joints

C. Genetic predisposition

D. Collagen overproduction

Q29. Following injury immediately, which phase of wound healing involves the initiation of coagulation and hemostasis?

A. Proliferation

B. Wound remodelling

C. Inflammation

D. Coagulation and haemostasis

Q30. In terms of wound healing, what is the primary long-term aim of coagulation and hemostasis?

A. To prevent infection

B. To promote angiogenesis

C. To provide a matrix for invading cells

D. To initiate inflammation

Q31. For changing a dressing on a clean and non-infected surgical wound, what is the recommended frequency?

A. Every 4 hours.

B. Once a day.

C. Every 48 hours.

D. Only when it becomes soiled.

Q32. Which intervention is appropriate for promoting wound healing when managing a patient with a venous leg ulcer?

A. Keeping the affected leg elevated.

B. Applying dry gauze dressings.

C. Massaging the wound site vigorously.

D. Encouraging prolonged standing.

Q33. When can non-sterile gloves be used during dressing changes for optimal wound healing

A. Immediately

B. After 48 hours

C. After 72 hours

D. Only for contaminated wounds

Q34. When involving caregivers, what is an essential aspect to consider in the wound care plan?

A. Disregarding caregiver concerns and preferences.

B. Ensuring caregivers have extensive medical training.

C. Recognizing the impact of caregivers on treatment outcomes.

D. Limiting communication with caregivers to minimize confusion.

Q35. While determining the financial feasibility of wound care supplies for a patient, what primary factor should be considered?

A. Recommending the most expensive options available.

B. Prioritizing products regardless of cost.

C. Ensuring reimbursement covers all expenses.

D. Selecting treatments within the patient's financial means.

Q36. In wound care planning, what is the importance of setting realistic goals?

A. Unrealistic goals enhance patient motivation.

B. Unrealistic goals can lead to treatment failure and non-adherence.

C. Unrealistic goals have no impact on treatment outcomes.

D. Unrealistic goals are essential to challenge patients.

Q37. The diagnostic test that provides a quantitative assessment of calf muscle pump function and calf venous reflux is:

A. Air plethysmography.

B. Photoplethysmography.

C. Doppler ultrasonography.

D. Contrast venogram.

Q38. What would be the role of concomitant chemotherapy if a patient undergoing combination therapy is at risk for severe radiation skin reactions?

A. Sensitizing basal cells to radiation

B. Reducing the risk of skin reactions

C. Enhancing functional outcome

D. Minimizing total radiation dose

Q39. In a patient with suspected arterial ulcers, what diagnostic test would be suitable if a healthcare provider needs to assess arterial waveforms?

A. Toe pressure measurements.

B. Doppler waveform analysis.

C. Transcutaneous oxygen measurements (TcPO2).

D. Skin perfusion pressure (SPP).

Q40. What is the primary purpose of lower-extremity angiography in a patient, suspected of having arterial ulcers?

A. Assessing arterial waveforms.

B. Determining toe-brachial index.

C. Diagnosing arterial vascular disease.

D. Evaluating microvascular circulation.

Q41. To assess arterial functioning noninvasively by measuring blood pressures at various sites on the lower extremities, which diagnostic test is performed?

A. Toe-brachial index measurement.

B. Lower-extremity angiography.

C. Color duplex scanning.

D. Segmental pressures assessment.

Q42. A healthcare provider is performing perfusion assessment tests like ABI and tissue perfusion testing in patients with suspected venous ulcers. What is the primary purpose of this procedure?

A. Assessing venous reflux severity.

B. Identifying patients for venous reconstruction.

C. Evaluating the presence of arterial insufficiency.

D. Determining wound healing potential.

Q43. In pressure ulcer development, what is the role of protein deficiency?

A. Increases oxygen diffusion

B. Enhances tissue regeneration

C. Decreases immune function

D. Promotes collagen synthesis

Q44. In acutely ill veterans, which medical factor has a stronger predictive value for pressure ulcer development?

A. Nutritional status

B. Mobility

C. Braden scale score

D. Pain level

Q45. What effect does the deficiency of vitamin A have on wound healing in a patient with a pressure ulcer?

A. Delays reepithelialization

B. Enhances collagen synthesis

C. Stabilizes cell membranes

D. Increases oxygen diffusion

Q46. The primary purpose of conducting a comprehensive nutrition assessment is:

A. To diagnose malnutrition.

B. To prescribe nutritional supplements.

C. To determine appropriate nutrition interventions.

D. To assess biochemical markers of nutrition.

Q47. Which mineral supplementation is most likely to improve collagen formation and phagocytic activity in a patient with anemia, exhibiting impaired wound healing due to chronic kidney disease?

A. Zinc

B. Iron

C. Copper

D. Magnesium

Q48. Signs of poor wound healing are found in a 60-year-old patient with a chronic wound on his lower leg despite standard care. A limited intake of protein-rich foods is revealed in his diet history. What nutritional intervention is most appropriate in this case?

A. Recommending protein supplementation

B. Advising increased carbohydrate intake

C. Suggesting fat-restricted diet

D. Encouraging vitamin C supplementation

Q49. What treatment approach is recommended for a patient's chronic wound, showing no systemic signs of infection but presenting with nonhealing, increased exudate and a malodorous smell?

A. Systemic antibiotics

B. Topical antimicrobials

C. Surgical debridement

D. Biofilm disruption

Q50. What complicating factor may contribute to muted or absent classic signs of wound infection in a patient's chronic wound, which presents with erythema, increased exudate, and a history of steroid therapy?

A. Poor wound hygiene

B. Immunocompromised status

C. Surgical history

D. Inadequate debridement

Q51. A chronic wound with a dry crust is observed by a wound care nurse. In this wound, what factor delays keratinocyte migration and epithelial resurfacing?

A. Moist wound environment

B. Matrix metalloproteinase secretion

C. Hypoxic wound conditions

D. Elevated bacteria levels

Q52. What bacterial burden seriously impairs wound healing for a patient who presents with a chronic wound showing signs of inflammation and bacterial colonization?

A. 10^4 organisms per gram of tissue

B. 10^5 organisms per gram of tissue

C. 10^6 organisms per gram of tissue

D. 10^7 organisms per gram of tissue

Q53. What is the gold standard debridement method for diabetic foot ulcers requiring debridement to stimulate healing?

A. Autolytic debridement

B. Surgical debridement

C. Enzymatic debridement

D. Sharp debridement

Q54. A wound care clinician employs the NPUAP/AHCPR system to assess a pressure ulcer. What is the limitation of this system in the context of assessing wound healing?

A. Lack of standardized assessment methods

B. Inability to determine the wound's healing stage

C. Reliance on acute wound healing models

D. Requirement for reverse staging during healing

Q55. What determines the severity of the injury and influences the choice of treatment in the context of burn wound treatment?

A. Age of the patient

B. Presence of electrical injury

C. Number of cells injured or destroyed

D. Surface area affected by the burn

Q56.What aspect should be assessed weekly and revised as necessary when developing a treatment plan for burn wounds?

A. Patient's age

B. Wound bed score

C. Presence of infection

D. Use of surgical intervention

Q57. A nurse is setting up HVPC treatment for a wound on the right hip, coccyx, left foot, and right heel. In this case, where should the dispersive electrode be placed to optimize current flow?

A. Over the right hip

B. Over the left thigh

C. Over the coccyx

D. Over the right heel

Q58. In the context of HVPC treatment, how should a dispersive electrode be positioned to achieve good contact with the skin and avoid bony prominences?

A. Place it directly over the wound

B. Use a plastic sheet under the electrode

C. Put it on the bed without securing

D. Position it proximal to the wound

Q59. A nurse is attempting surgical closure for venous ulcers. What should be done before this procedure to ensure minimal bacterial levels and no beta-hemolytic streptococci in the wound?

A. Administer systemic antibiotics

B. Apply antiseptic dressings

C. Use prophylactic wound irrigation

D. Minimize tissue bacterial load

Q60. What is crucial for minimizing factors that increase the risk of ulceration and amputation for a diabetic patient who participates in a general diabetes self-management program?

A. Daily foot examinations

B. Weekly foot massages

C. Monthly pedicures

D. Yearly podiatrist visits

Q61. In the context of facilitating diabetes self-management, what is the key advice for a healthcare professional?

A. Maintain a directive style

B. Adopt a collaborative interactive style

C. Rely on comprehensive programs

D. Avoid involving patients in defining treatment goals

Q62. What factor might require continual surveillance by an expert when a caregiver struggles to manage a patient's malignant wound?

A. Odor control techniques

B. Wound appearance changes

C. Increased fluid intake

D. Patient's emotional distress

Q63. What contributes to the goal of satisfactory psychological well-being when educating caregivers on managing malignant cutaneous wounds?

A. Complete wound healing

B. Achieving unrealistic goals

C. Alleviating pain and managing symptoms

D. Ignoring changes in wound appearance

Q64. What principle guides the management of wound bioburden when a patient's chronic wound exhibits delayed healing and friable granulation tissue?

A. Minimize cofactors

B. Provide optimal wound environment

C. Eliminate or reduce causative factors

D. Topical antimicrobial therapy

Q65. What is crucial for the administration to demand regarding the educational preparation of healthcare professionals when developing a skin and wound management program?

A. Attendance at individual seminars

B. Completion of continuing education courses

C. Appropriate education, qualifications, and credentialing

D. Collection of certificates of completion

Q66. There is a patient with peripheral vascular disease. The patient is at risk for ulcerations. In this situation, what area within treatment field is particularly susceptible to severe reactions?

A. Bony prominences

B. Skin folds

C. Axillae

D. Neck

Q67. There is a patient with suspected venous ulcers. The patient requires quantitative assessment of calf venous reflux. In this case, which diagnostic test should be performed to determine the best course of treatment?

A. Contrast venogram

B. Doppler ultrasonography

C. Photoplethysmography

D. Ankle-brachial index (ABI)

Q68. What is the critical aspect for wound healing, limb salvage, and long-term survival to reduce the risk of lead-related arterial disease (LEAD)?

A. Avoiding lifestyle modifications

B. Managing underlying disease processes

C. Irreversible risk factors

D. Emphasizing family history

Q69.In the context of minimizing the risk, what should the patients with potential lymphedema be aware of?

A. Delayed appearance of lymphedema after a causative event

B. Avoiding contact with healthcare professionals

C. Wearing tight clothing and accessories

D. Not seeking medical attention for early signs and symptoms

Q70. Which of the following interventions help identify triggers and manage triggering events for tobacco users?

A. Avoidance of stress management

B. Prescribing nicotine replacement therapy

C. Appropriate use of compression stockings

D. Anticipatory guidance counseling

Q71. Which of the following is a modifiable factor that contributes to LEAD progression?

A. Family history

B. Advanced age

C. Elevated homocysteine levels

D. Inactivity

Q72. In patients with pressure ulcers, what is the significance of vitamin C deficiency?

A. Enhances collagen synthesis

B. Aids in fat metabolism

C. Stabilizes cell membranes

D. Increases oxygen diffusion

Q73. What is the recommended strategy for reducing SSI risk in patients undergoing elective surgery?

A. Ritualistic behavior

B. Antimicrobial stewardship

C. Extended surgery duration

D. Inadequate surgical closure

Q74. Which of the following methods is most recommended for accurately tracking healing progress in a patient with a chronic wound?

A. Verbal descriptions in the patient's chart

B. Utilizing standardized forms for documentation

C. Serial photographs of the wound

D. Regular measurements with a ruler

Q75. Which method can be effectively promoted when a wound care facility wants to ensure consistency and completeness in wound documentation?

A. Verbal descriptions during team meetings

B. Using various terminology for diversity

C. Utilizing standardized forms for documentation

D. Avoiding documentation altogether

Q76. Why tunneling measurements are not part of the Pressure Ulcer Scale for Healing?

A. Lack of clinical practicality

B. Inaccuracy in measuring tunneling

C. No impact on validity and reliability

D. Difficulty in documenting tunneling

Q77. A patient with a venous leg ulcer should be educated on:

A. Elevation of the affected limb.

B. Applying heat to promote circulation.

C. Massaging the ulcer to reduce swelling.

D. Avoiding compression therapy.

Q78. A patient presents with a stage 2 pressure injury on their sacrum. What characteristic defines a stage 2 pressure injury?

A. Full-thickness skin loss

B. Non-blanch-able erythema

C. Exposed adipose tissue

D. Visible muscle or bone

Q79. A patient with a stage 4 pressure ulcer on the heel should be repositioned:

A. Every 2 hours.

B. Every 4 hours.

C. Every 6 hours.

D. Once a day.

Q80. A patient with a diabetic foot ulcer is discharged home with instructions for self-care. The nurse should emphasize:

A. Avoiding daily foot inspection.

B. Wearing tight-fitting shoes.

C. Moisturizing the feet daily.

D. Avoid walking barefoot.

Q81. For accurate wound care documentation, which component is crucial?

A. Patient demographics

B. Wound assessment details

C. Treatment plan specifics

D. Progress notes recording

Q82. In wound management, why is collaboration with other healthcare providers important?

A. To enhance patient education

B. To improve communication

C. To ensure continuity of care

D. To facilitate progress notes recording

Q83. What is identified as a potential barrier to the success of a project aimed at improving wound care practices in a healthcare facility that amalgamates?

A. Presence of quality improvement activities

B. Lack of coordination across sites

C. Autonomy of individual facilities

D. Absence of professional innovators

Q84. What percentage of audited clinical areas had guidelines ensuring information-guided nursing interventions to address the clinical management gap?

A. Over 50%

B. Exactly 50%

C. Less than 50%

D. No clinical areas had guidelines.

Q85. How did the wound care program ensure the relevance of guidelines across the care continuum, including general practitioners and community care?

A. By restricting access to guidelines.

B. Developing one-page policy summaries.

C. Excluding general practitioners.

D. Avoiding community care involvement.

Q86. Considering the following options, what is the key principle underlying the adaptation of wound care policies by local committees?

A. Strict adherence to centralized decisions.

B. Local adaptation fosters user acceptance.

C. Users' resistance to change is essential.

D. Avoiding any adaptation to maintain uniformity.

Q87. What legal precautions should a physician take when a patient returns with symptoms of infection after suturing a wound?

A. Provide no further treatment

B. Obtain informed consent for surgery

C. Document the post-surgical care plan

D. Prescribe antibiotics and document accordingly

Q88. What legal concept should a physician uphold when a patient presents with a wound and requests immediate surgery?

A. Patient autonomy

B. Therapeutic privilege

C. Standard of care

D. Informed refusal

Q89. What percentage of lacerations caused by glass is reported to have retained foreign bodies?

A. 2%

B. 5%

C. 7%

D. 10%

Q90. What is the nurse's first action when a postoperative patient develops serosanguinous drainage from a surgical incision?

A. Apply a sterile dressing.

B. Notify the healthcare provider.

C. Document the finding.

D. Increase the frequency of dressing changes.

Q91. When a patient with a chronic venous leg ulcer asks about dietary recommendations. The nurse's best advice is to:

A. Increase protein intake.

B. Limit sodium consumption.

C. Consume more carbohydrates.

D. Follow a high-fat diet.

Q92. During palpation of a wound, a post-surgical patient reports pain. What aspect should the nurse specifically assess?

A. Skin color

B. Lesion size

C. Texture

D. Bruising

Q93. In the skin assessment of a patient with a history of falls and skin lesions with vascularity changes, what extrinsic factor should be considered?

A. Immobility

B. Accidents

C. Pressure

D. Surgical procedures

Q94. How does dehydration affect wound healing in a patient with compromised skin integrity has reduced fluid intake?

A. Enhances cell metabolism

B. Preserves cell structure

C. Disturbs cell metabolism and wound healing

D. Accelerates tissue regeneration

Q95. How often should skin inspections occur for high-risk patients when a caregiver in a long-term care facility is instructed to assess an immobile patient's skin integrity?

A. Daily

B. Weekly

C. Monthly

D. Once per shift

Q96. Which of the following layers of the epidermis acts as a waterproof barrier that protects against infectious microorganisms and environmental elements?

A. Stratum basale

B. Stratum granulosum

C. Stratum corneum

D. Stratum lucidum

Q97. A patient with age-related skin changes, including reduced subcutaneous fat, is at increased risk for:

A. excessive sebum production.

B. impaired thermoregulation.

C. heightened sensitivity to sunlight.

D. improved resistance to skin breakdown.

Q98. Which skin condition is likely to occur in a patient with a compromised epidermal lipid barrier?

A. Dry, flaky skin.

B. Increased melanin production.

C. Excessive sebum secretion.

D. Elevated stratum corneum thickness.

Q99. A patient with diabetic neuropathy experiences microvascular damage contributing to peripheral neuropathy. The underlying process of microvascular damage is most effectively addressed by:

A. Lowering HbA1c levels.

B. Using prostacyclins.

C. Gene therapy interventions.

D. Hyperbaric oxygen therapy.

Q100. A patient with atopic dermatitis (eczema) and persistent dry, itchy skin seeks relief. The most suitable treatment approach involves:

A. Topical corticosteroids.

B. Antihistamines.

C. Emollients and moisturizers.

D. Systemic antibiotics.

Q101. A patient with peripheral arterial disease (PAD) and a non-healing foot ulcer is at risk of amputation. What factor significantly impairs wound healing in PAD patients with diabetes?

A. Neuropathy

B. Infection

C. Ischemia

D. Edema

Q102. A clinician is assessing wound bed preparation for a venous stasis ulcer. What does the Wound Bed Score (WBS) evaluate to determine the likelihood of wound closure?

A. Color of the wound bed

B. Presence of eschar

C. Fibrinous material

D. Surrounding skin condition

Q103. A patient with a venous leg ulcer undergoes healing through secondary intention. What is the main process involved in this type of wound healing?

A. Epithelization

B. Granulation and epithelization

C. Maturation

D. Proliferation

Q104. A patient's wound is in the proliferative phase of wound healing. Which cell type is primarily responsible for the regeneration of new tissue and blood vessels during this phase?

A. Macrophages

B. Fibroblasts

C. Platelets

D. White blood cells

Q105. A patient with delayed wound closure lacks skin gamma-delta T-cells. What is the specific role of skin gamma-delta T-cells in wound healing?

A. Inducing apoptosis

B. Regulating inflammation

C. Supporting keratinocyte proliferation

D. Stimulating angiogenesis

Q106. Which cell type is involved in wound-induced hypoxia and contributes significantly to neovascularization in the wound-healing process?

A. Neutrophils

B. Macrophages

C. Epidermal stem cells

D. Endothelial progenitor cells

Q107. What is hyperbaric oxygen therapy's (HBOT) role in potentially overcoming tissue hypoxia in wound healing?

A. Inducing hyperoxia

B. Reducing oxidative stress

C. Enhancing cytokine production

D. Promoting collagen synthesis

Q108. What role does oxygen play in the process of wound healing?

A. Inhibits angiogenesis

B. Suppresses fibroblast proliferation

C. Delays re-epithelialization

D. Supports collagen synthesis and fibroblast proliferation

Q109. What is the contribution of peripheral vascular disease (PAD) to delayed wound healing and the development of chronic, ischemic ulcers?

A. Increased blood flow

B. Enhanced tissue perfusion

C. Stenosis and narrowing of blood vessels

D. Rapid healing response

Q110. Why is it crucial to detect and screen for peripheral vascular disease (PAD) early for limb salvage?

A. To prevent chronic inflammation

B. To limit tissue edema

C. To avoid amputations

D. To expedite wound healing

Test 2 Answer Key

Q1.

Answer: D.

Explanation: For confirming arterial insufficiency in patients with suspected (PAD), contrast arteriography is recognized as the gold standard diagnostic test, providing detailed images of arterial blood flow.

Q2.

Answer: C

Explanation: In the management of diabetic foot wounds and detecting peripheral arterial disease, the assessment of blood flow and vascular status through ABI is crucial.

Q3.

Answer: B.

Explanation: High-protein diets facilitate tissue repair and regeneration, thereby aiding the healing process in diabetic ulcers. It is essential for individuals to uphold sufficient protein intake to promote effective wound healing.

Q4.

Answer: D.

Explanation: Considering the contraindications associated with sustained compression in patients with compromised cardiac function, it is crucial to completely assess the patient's cardiac history and signs of heart failure before initiating compression therapy.

Q5.

Answer: C.

Explanation: Ensuring optimal wound healing outcomes and addressing malnutrition in patients with diabetic foot ulcers requires collaboration with a registered dietitian for nutritional assessment and intervention.

Q6.

Answer: C

Explanation: Supporting wound healing and preventing foot ulcers in diabetic patients necessitates adequate protein intake. Maintaining tissue integrity and promoting recovery is significantly facilitated by adequate protein consumption.

Q7.

Answer: D

Explanation: Facilitating wound closure and tissue repair, adequate zinc intake is essential for wound healing as it plays a critical role in collagen synthesis, immune function, and epithelialization.

Q8.

Answer: A

Explanation: The utilization of a pain questionnaire is crucial for guiding appropriate pain management strategies by determining the pain pattern, intensity, and type, thereby facilitating a structured assessment.

Q9.

Answer: C.

Explanation: Considering pertinent familial tendencies and personal health records aids healthcare providers in understanding the patient's past medical issues, facilitating targeted interventions, and elucidating potential etiologies of limb swelling.

Q10.

Answer: B.

Explanation: Surgical intervention is often necessary at this advanced stage of stage 4 pressure injuries, especially for removing necrotic tissue and facilitating healing, particularly for addressing deep tissue damage and encouraging recovery.

Q11.

Answer: A.

Explanation: Pale, cool skin characterizes arterial insufficiency due to reduced blood flow to the extremities, indicating compromised circulation, which can lead to various complications in the absence of treatment.

Q12.

Answer: B.

Explanation: In promoting wound healing, enzymatic debridement agents facilitate the removal of necrotic tissue. While silver dressings may have antimicrobial properties but will not assist in debridement.

Q13.

Answer: B

Explanation: The primary purpose of hydrocolloid dressings is to keep wounds moist, fostering ideal conditions for effective healing. They facilitate tissue repair and regeneration by creating a supportive environment that aids in the healing process.

Q14.

Answer: D

Explanation: Preventing hindrance of the healing process and facilitating optimal wound healing requires controlling excessive exudate in wounds.

Q15.

Answer: B

Explanation: In promoting a clean wound bed and supporting the body's natural healing mechanisms, mechanical debridement is essential for slough removal, aiding in wound healing. This process is necessary to clear away dead tissue.

Q16.

Answer: A

Explanation: Typically found on pressure points due to poor circulation, arterial ulcers often cause intense pain, particularly at night.

Q17.

Answer: C

Explanation: Prolonged exposure to urinary or fecal incontinence commonly leads to moisture-associated skin damage (MASD) in palliative care patients, resulting in skin breakdown.

Q18.

Answer: B

Explanation: Characterized by the production and placement of extracellular matrix proteins, fibroplasia represents the tissue repair phase, crucial for tissue regeneration and wound closure, with cells producing structural elements.

Q19.

Answer: B

Explanation: Commonly associated with conditions like diabetes and long-term smoking, gangrene is marked by tissue decay due to poor blood supply.

Q20.

Answer: D

Explanation: If severe or complicated, traumatic wounds disrupt normal tissue architecture and may fail to heal within expected timeframes.

Q21.

Answer: A

Explanation: While open wounds have damaged skin exposing underlying tissue, closed wounds involve trauma to underlying tissue without breaking the skin.

Q22.

Answer: A

Explanation: Aiding in determining appropriate interventions and monitoring healing progress, digital palpation of the wound bed helps assess tissue depth and extent of involvement.

Q23.

Answer: A

Explanation: Tissue displacement and potential undermining occur as a result of shear injuries, which arise from the interplay of gravity and friction inducing opposing motions of tissue layers, elucidating their etiological underpinnings.

Q24.

Answer: D.

Explanation: Underscoring the unique regenerative capacity observed in fetal tissues compared to adults, fetal wound healing features high levels of HA, facilitating scarless repair, unlike adult wound healing.

Q25.

Answer: A.

Explanation: Collagen III plays a crucial role in enhancing wound strength and structural integrity by transforming into collagen I during maturation. This conversion process is essential for effective healing of damaged tissue.

Q26.

Answer: A

Explanation: During the initial stages of the inflammation, neutrophils serve as initial scavengers for debridement, phagocytizing dead tissue and creating a hostile environment for bacteria.

Q27.

Answer: A

Explanation: By contributing to the initiation of wound repair processes, interleukin, released by neutrophils during the inflammatory phase, acts as a proinflammatory cytokine and stimulates the proliferation of keratinocytes.

Q28.

Answer: A

Explanation: Hyperelastic skin is a common manifestation of Ehlers-Danlos syndrome caused by collagen abnormalities, which may lead to slower wound healing. The characteristic features of the syndrome, including skin fragility and impaired tissue repair, arise from these inherent collagen defects.

Q29.

Answer: D.

Explanation: To control bleeding and initiate the repair process, the initial phase of wound healing is coagulation and hemostasis, which begins immediately after injury.

Q30.

Answer: C

Explanation: While facilitating tissue repair and regeneration, coagulation and haemostasis aim to provide a matrix for invading cells in the later phases of healing.

Q31.

Answer: D

Explanation: To prevent infection without disrupting the wound's healing process and maintain a clean environment, dressings should be changed when soiled.

Q32.

Answer: A

Explanation: Edema and venous pressure are reduced by elevating the affected leg. This aids in ulcer healing.

Q33.

Answer: B

Explanation: In wound healing, non-sterile gloves can be used for dressing changes with primary intention after 48 hours. Minimizing unnecessary barrier use promotes the aseptic technique.

Q34.

Answer: C

Explanation: Involving caregivers enhances the likelihood of treatment success and acknowledges their significant role.

Q35.

Answer: D

Explanation: Selecting treatments within the patient's financial means promotes patient adherence and ensures continuity of care.

Q36.

Answer: B

Explanation: While preventing disappointment and treatment failure, realistic goals promote patient confidence and adherence.

Q37.

Answer: A

Explanation: Air plethysmography determines suitability for venous reconstruction and venous disease severity, and measures the venous filling index.

Q38.

Answer: A

Explanation: In patients undergoing combination therapy, concomitant chemotherapy may sensitize basal cells to radiation which increases the risk of severe skin reactions.

Q39.

Answer: B

Explanation: Doppler waveform analysis indicates moderate arterial occlusive disease with a monophasic waveform and provides valuable information about arterial waveforms.

Q40.

Answer: C

Explanation: In patients with suspected arterial ulcers, lower-extremity angiography is the gold standard for confirming the diagnosis.

Q41.

Answer: D

Explanation: By recording blood pressures at different sites on the lower extremities, Segmental pressure assessment measures arterial functioning noninvasively.

Q42.

Answer: C

Explanation: In patients with suspected venous ulcers, the primary purpose of perfusion assessment tests like ABI and tissue perfusion testing is to evaluate the presence of arterial insufficiency.

Q43.

Answer: C

Explanation: Immune function is decreased by protein deficiency. It makes tissues more susceptible to breakdown and pressure ulcer development.

Q44.

Answer: A

Explanation: For pressure ulcer development, nutritional status has a stronger predictive value than Braden scale scores alone along with other medical factors.

Q45.

Answer: A

Explanation: The deficiency of vitamin A impairs wound healing by delaying reepithelialization, collagen synthesis, and cellular cohesion.

Q46.

Answer: C

Explanation: Determining the appropriate nutrition interventions based on gathered data is the primary purpose of a comprehensive nutrition assessment.

Q47.

Answer: B

Explanation: Iron is essential for oxygen transport, effective wound healing, and crucial for hemoglobin production.

Q48.

Answer: A

Explanation: To promote wound healing, protein supplementation is crucial particularly in patients with inadequate protein intake.

Q49.

Answer: B

Explanation: To effectively manage microbial bioburden, topical antimicrobial treatment is recommended for wounds, exhibiting signs of critical colonization.

Q50.

Answer: B

Explanation: Immunocompromised status can impair the inflammatory response like from steroid therapy. This leads to muted or absent classic signs of wound infection.

Q51.

Answer: D

Explanation: Elevated bacteria levels delay wound healing, promote the formation of a dry crust, and inhibit keratinocyte migration and epithelial resurfacing.

Q52.

Answer: C

Explanation: A bacterial burden of 10^6 organisms or more per gram of tissue necessitates aggressive treatment. This bacterial burden seriously impairs wound healing.

Q53.

Answer: D

Explanation: Sharp debridement removes necrotic tissue and stimulates healing effectively. It is considered the gold standard method for debridement in diabetic foot ulcers.

Q54.

Answer: C

Explanation: The NPUAP/AHCPR system may not follow the linear progression of acute healing phases. It is developed for acute wounds and is not suitable for assessing wound healing in chronic wounds.

Q55.

Answer: C

Explanation: The depth of the burn injury is based on the number of cells injured or destroyed. It determines the severity and guides the treatment approach.

Q56.

Answer: B

Explanation: Wound bed score should be assessed weekly and revised when developing a treatment plan for burn wounds. The wound bed score is regularly evaluated to ensure the burn wound is appropriately prepared for effective treatment.

Q57.

Answer: B

Explanation: Placing the dispersive electrode over the left thigh benefits the wounds on the right hip, coccyx, left foot, and right heel. This technique also optimizes current flow through deep tissues.

Q58.

Answer: D

Explanation: The dispersive electrode should be placed proximal to the wound over soft tissues. This technique ensures good contact and avoids bony prominences.

Q59.

Answer: D

Explanation: Minimizing tissue bacterial levels to ≤ 105 CFU/g before surgical closure is crucial. This step avoids beta-hemolytic streptococci in venous ulcers for successful closure.

Q60.

Answer: A

Explanation: Patients must understand the importance of daily foot examinations and take appropriate measures to reduce ulceration and amputation risk.

Q61.

Answer: B

Explanation: Successful diabetes self-management requires a collaborative approach. This approach involves patients defining problems, goals, and management strategies for better outcomes.

Q62.

Answer: B

Explanation: Wound appearance changes and complicated pouching techniques might require continual surveillance and enhance care for patients with malignant wounds.

Q63.

Answer: C

Explanation: Alleviating pain and managing symptoms enhance the quality of life for patients with malignant cutaneous Wounds. This process contributes to satisfactory psychological well-being.

Q64.

Answer: A

Explanation: To manage wound bioburden effectively, minimizing cofactors, such as addressing nutritional deficiencies, is essential alongside topical antimicrobial therapy.

Q65.

Answer: C

Explanation: It is crucial for the administration to demand appropriate education, qualifications, and credentialing for healthcare professionals involved in skin and wound management programs.

Q66.

Answer: B

Explanation: In patients with peripheral vascular disease, moist areas on the body, such as skin folds, are at risk for severe reactions, emphasizing preventive strategies.

Q67.

Answer: B

Explanation: Doppler ultrasonography guides the treatment decisions and optimize patient outcomes. It provides accurate assessment of calf venous reflux.

Q68.

Answer: B

Explanation: Effectively managing underlying disease processes is critical for wound healing, limb salvage, and long-term survival to reduce the risk of lead-related arterial disease (LEAD).

Q69.

Answer: A

Explanation: Patients with potential lymphedema should be aware of the delayed appearance of lymphedema after a causative event, emphasizing the importance of monitoring for early signs and symptoms.

Q70.

Answer: D

Explanation: Anticipatory guidance counselling helps to identify triggers and manage triggering events for tobacco users. It provides valuable support to individuals attempting tobacco cessation.

Q71.

Answer: D

Explanation: Inactivity is a modifiable factor that significantly contributes to the progression of LEAD. This factor emphasizes the importance of lifestyle modifications.

Q72.

Answer: A

Explanation: Vitamin C deficiency enhances collagen synthesis and contributes to poor wound healing in patients with pressure ulcers.

Q73.

Answer: B

Explanation: Pre-operative assessment and evidence-based practices enhance outcomes. Patients undergoing elective surgery are recommended strategies aligned with antimicrobial stewardship practices to reduce SSI risk.

Q74.

Answer: C

Explanation: The most recommended method for accurately tracking the healing progress of a patient with a chronic wound is serial photographs of the wound. It provides a permanent record of wound progression.

Q75.

Answer: C

Explanation: The utilization of standardized forms can effectively promote consistency and completeness in wound documentation.

Q76.

Answer: C

Explanation: Tunneling measurements were excluded from the Pressure Ulcer Scale for Healing as they did not improve the tool's validity and reliability. Inclusion in the Pressure Ulcer Scale for Healing should be decided by facilities based on clinical needs.

Q77.

Answer: A

Explanation: Elevation aids in reducing edema and improving venous return, essential for managing venous leg ulcers effectively.

Q78.

Answer: B

Explanation: Stage 2 pressure injuries involve partial-thickness loss of skin with non-blanchable erythema.

Q79.

Answer: A

Explanation: Frequent repositioning minimizes pressure and shear forces, aiding in pressure ulcer prevention and management.

Q80.

Answer: D

Explanation: Walking barefoot increases the risk of injury and infection in patients with diabetic foot ulcers, so it should be avoided.

Q81.

Answer: B

Explanation: Wound assessment details are crucial for accurate wound care documentation by providing essential information for treatment planning and monitoring.

Q82.

Answer: C

Explanation: Collaboration promotes comprehensive patient management and better outcomes. It ensures a multidisciplinary approach to wound care.

Q83.

Answer: C

Explanation: The autonomy of individual facilities is identified as a potential barrier to the success of the project, emphasizing the importance of coordination and standardization.

Q84.

Answer: C

Explanation: Less than 50% of audited clinical areas had guidelines ensuring information-guided nursing interventions to address the clinical management gap.

Q85.

Answer: B

Explanation: The wound care program ensures the relevance of guidelines across the care continuum by developing one-page policy summaries.

Q86.

Answer: B

Explanation: Local adaptation aligns with the principle that people resent changes imposed on them but not decisions they have contributed to. It ensures user involvement and acceptance.

Q87.

Answer: D

Explanation: Prescribing antibiotics and documenting care mitigate legal risk in cases of post-surgical infection.

Q88.

Answer: A

Explanation: Respecting patient autonomy entails informing patients of their treatment options and obtaining their informed consent.

Q89.

Answer: C

Explanation: Approximately 7% of lacerations caused by glass are reported to have retained foreign bodies.

Q90.

Answer: C

Explanation: The first action is to document the serosanguinous drainage to provide an accurate record of the wound status before proceeding with further actions.

Q91.

Answer: B

Explanation: The nurse's best advice is to limit sodium intake because it helps manage edema associated with venous leg ulcers and promotes better wound-healing outcomes.

Q92.

Answer: C

Explanation: During palpation assessing texture helps identify pain associated with the wound. This information is crucial for tailoring pain management strategies and implementing wound care interventions.

Q93.

Answer: B

Explanation: In the skin assessment, accidents, an extrinsic factor, should be considered when a patient with a history of falls has skin lesions with vascularity changes. Recognizing and addressing the external causes are essential for effective wound management.

Q94.

Answer: C

Explanation: By limiting the availability of essential nutrients and oxygen to the wound tissues, dehydration disturbs cell metabolism and wound healing. To support blood flow, prevent additional breakdown of the skin, and promote optimal wound healing, adequate fluid intake is important.

Q95.

Answer: D

Explanation: A proactive approach of once per shift allows for the early identification of skin issues, facilitating timely interventions to prevent complications like pressure injuries. High-risk patients, especially those with limited mobility, require frequent skin inspection at least once per shift.

Q96.

Answer: C

Explanation: The Stratum corneum is the outermost layer of the epidermis which acts as a waterproof barrier, safeguarding the skin against infections and environmental assaults.

Q97.

Answer: B

Explanation: The reduction in impaired thermoregulation in natural insulation elevates the risk of skin breakdown, emphasizing the importance of preventive measures. Diminished subcutaneous fat, characteristic of age-related changes, increases vulnerability to impaired thermoregulation.

Q98.

Answer: A

Explanation: Dry, flaky skin emphasizes the significance of maintaining lipid integrity for optimal skin health. A deficient epidermal lipid barrier leads to increased transepidermal water loss, resulting in dry, flaky skin.

Q99.

Answer: A

Explanation: Lowering HbA1c levels has been shown to decrease microvascular damage associated with diabetic neuropathy, addressing the underlying process and promoting nerve health.

Q100.

Answer: C

Explanation: Emollients and moisturizers play a crucial role in managing atopic dermatitis, providing relief from dry, itchy skin and preventing exacerbations.

Q101.

Answer: C

Explanation: In PAD patients with diabetes, inadequate tissue perfusion due to ischemia significantly hinders wound healing.

Q102.

Answer: D

Explanation: The WBS considers surrounding skin factors, including healing edges and periwound dermatitis, to predict wound closure likelihood.

Q103.

Answer: B

Explanation: Secondary intention healing in venous leg ulcers involves granulation and epithelization, akin to the process of rebuilding a house after a fire.

Q104.

Answer: B

Explanation: Fibroblasts are the key cells in the proliferative phase, contributing to the regeneration of new tissue, blood vessels, and connective tissue.

Q105.

Answer: B

Explanation: Skin gamma-delta T-cells regulate inflammation, contribute to tissue integrity, and play a role in wound healing by producing growth factors supporting keratinocyte proliferation.

Q106.

Answer: D

Explanation: Endothelial progenitor cells derived from the hematopoietic stem cell lineage play a significant role in neovascularization during wound-induced hypoxia.

Q107.

Answer: A

Explanation: HBOT overcome tissue hypoxia and supports wound healing processes by inducing a state of hyperoxia. Hyperbaric oxygen therapy (HBOT) increases oxygen levels.

Q108.

Answer: D

Explanation: Oxygen promotes optimal healing conditions. It is crucial for wound healing processes, including collagen synthesis and fibroblast proliferation.

Q109.

Answer: C

Explanation: PAD leads to stenosis and vessel narrowing. It reduces blood flow, causing delayed wound healing and promoting the development of chronic, ischemic ulcers.

Q110.

Answer: C

Explanation: Early detection and screening of peripheral vascular disease (PAD) is crucial to prevent lower limb amputations because compromised blood flow in PAD leads to delayed wound healing.

Rewards

Here are the three amazing rewards for my readers: -

1. **Audio File**

   Audio file of 2 Practice test in MP3 Format

2. **Flash Cards**

   200 Flash Cards in Anki app Format

3. **Extra Practice test**

   1 Extra Practice test in PDF file format

Please Scan QR below to get these rewards

Made in the USA
Monee, IL
26 October 2024

68691997R00052